GW00499867

Instant Vortex
Air Fryer Oven
Snacks Cookbook

DELICIOUS AND EASY TO MAKE
HEALTHY SNACKS RECIPES
IN YOUR AIR FRYER OVEN

VICTORIA SKINN

1

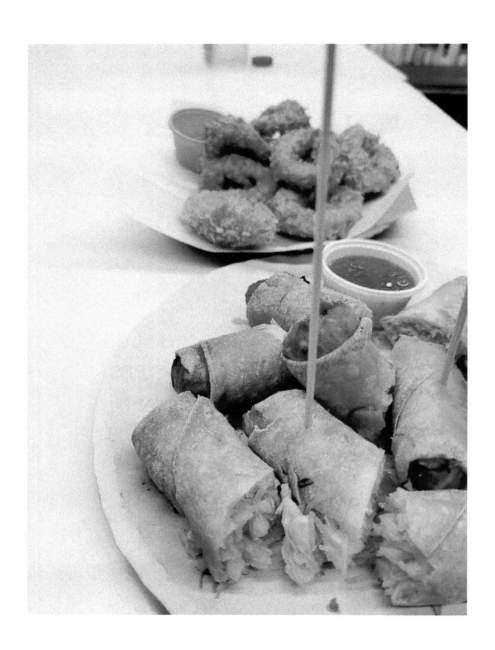

Table of contents

Introduction

The Instant Vortex Air Fryer Oven is an "all-in-one" kitchen appliance that promises **to replace a deep fryer, convection oven and microwave**; it also lets you sauté your foods. The Instant Vortex Air Fryer Oven is a unique kitchen gadget designed to fry food in a special chamber using super-heated air. The hot air circulates inside the cooking chamber using the convection mechanism, cooking your food evenly from all sides. It uses the so-called Maillard effect – a chemical reaction that gives fried food that distinctive flavor. Thanks to the hot air, your food gets that crispy exterior and a moist interior and does not taste like the fat.

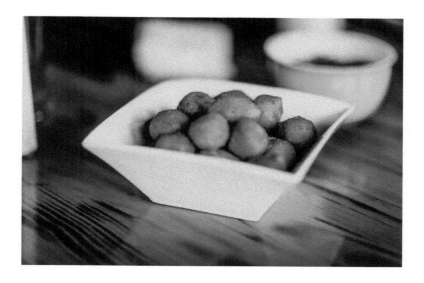

Why use an Air Fryer? I've been asked this question so many times, and my answer is always the same: it all boils down to versatility, **health**, and **speed**. It means that you can "set it and forget it" until it is done. Unlike most cooking methods, there's no need to keep an eye on it. **You can pick the ingredients, turn the machine on and walk away** – no worries about overcooked or burned food. Another great benefit of using an Air Fryer is that unlike the heat in an oven or on a stovetop, the heat in the cooking chamber is constant and it will cook your food evenly. Plus, it is energy-efficient and a space-saving solution.

Air fryers operate by cooking food with the flow of hot air. This is what makes the foods you put into it so crunchy when they come out!

Benefits of the Air Fryer

There are numerous benefits you'll get from using an Air Fryer. Here are the top three benefits of using an Air Fryer.

Fast cooking and convenience. The Instant Vortex Air Fryer Oven is an electric device, so you just need to press the right buttons and go about your business. It heats up in a few minutes so it can cut down cooking time; further, hot air circulates around your food, cooking it quickly and evenly. **Roast chicken is perfectly cooked in 30 minutes, baby back ribs in less than 25 minutes and beef chuck or steak in about 15 minutes**. You can use dividers and cook different foods at the same time. The Air Fryer is a real game-changer, it is a cost-saving solution in many ways. I also use my Air Fryer to keep my food warm. Air Fryer features include automatic temperature control, eliminating the need to slave over a hot stove.

Healthy eating. Yes, there is such a thing as healthy fried food and the Air Fryer proves that! The Air Fryer inspires me every day so that I enjoy cooking healthy and well-balanced meals for my family. Recent studies have shown that **air-fried foods contain up to 80% less fat in comparison to foods that are deep-fried**. Deep-fried food contributes to obesity, type 2 diabetes, high cholesterol, increased risk of heart disease, and so on. Plus, fats and oils become harmful under the high heat, which leads to increased inflammation in your body and speeds up aging. Further, these oils release cancer-causing toxic chemicals. Moreover, the spills of fats and oils injure wildlife and produce other undesirable effects on the planet Earth.

According to the leading experts, **you should not be afraid of healthy fats and oils, especially if you follow the ketogenic diet.** Avoid partially hydrogenated and genetically modified oils such as cottonseed oil, soybean oil, corn oil, and rice bran oil. You should also avoid margarine since it is loaded with trans-fats. Good fats and oils include olive oil, coconut oil, avocado oil, sesame oil, nuts and seeds. **Air-fried foods are delicious and have the texture of regular fried food, but they do not taste like fat.** French fries are only the beginning. Perfect ribs, hearty casseroles, fast snacks, and delectable desserts turn out great in this revolutionary kitchen gadget. When it comes to healthy dieting that does not compromise flavor, the Air Fryer is a real winner.

The ultimate solution to losing pounds and maintain a healthy weight. One of the greatest benefits of owning an Air Fryer is **the possibility to maintain an ideal weight in an easy and healthy way.** It doesn't mean that you must give up fried fish fillets, saucy steaks, and scrumptious desserts. Choosing a healthy-cooking technique is the key to success. Air frying requires less fat compared to many other cooking methods, making your weight loss diet more achievable.

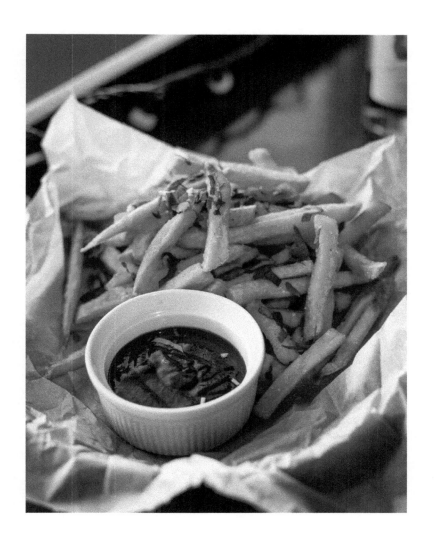

Understanding
Instant Vortex Air Fryer Oven

With the new generation of air fryer technology, one will enjoy crispy, guilt-free food. The Instant Vortex was created with many of the most critical features in mind: amazingly fast cooking times, a greater size, ease of cleaning, and basic, user-friendly settings. Instant Pot's popular smart system technology is used in the Instant Vortex to ensure the best performance every time. The sleek interface takes up very little counter space, and the intuitive touch screen and dial functions make it a joy to use. The Instant Vortex infuses your kitchen with a refreshing change. Enjoy the deep-fried taste, with the health advantages of air-frying and the dependability and comfort of a multifunctional gadget. One can air-fry, broil, roast, bake, dehydrate, reheat, and rotisserie the food with only one appliance.

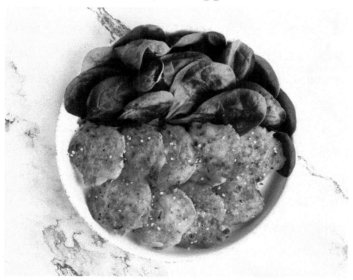

Instant vortex Air frying uses incredibly heating circulating air instead of hot oil to achieve the same crunchy, browned flavour and feel as deep-fried cuisine. It also traps moisture within the crispy crust, and it does so without any drawbacks of deep-frying: it's faster, safer, better, and requires less work. Instant vortex Air fryers are often much more flexible than deep fryers, limited to a single-use. Air frying allows one to barbecue a burger, roast tomatoes or a chicken, bake a pie or dehydrate fruit, and crisp up everything, from fritters to falafels and French fries… and many more! Do you like doughnuts? Or do you prefer Spicy & crispy wings? You may also make those. It's fine if the food is frozen, it is not necessary to thaw it first. Right from the fridge, nuggets have never tasted better.

What does it do?

The Instant Vortex's Air Fryer lets you make healthy versions of all their favourite fried foods, from natural to frozen, that are cooked to perfection and guilt-free. By using less oil you will get the deep-fried flavour and feel. It is easy to clean since less oil means less mess. The Vortex's Air Fryer uses hot circulating air rather than hot oil to provide the exact crunchy flavour and feel of deep-fried perfection. Air fried, grill, toast, and reheat in a flash with the pre-programmed Smart Programs. Juicy chicken wings, crispy potatoes, onion rings, and more are all air fried. Cauliflower bites, garlicky peas, chicken nuggets and shrimp skewers roast in the air fryer. Calzones, pizzas, soft cinnamon rolls and chewy brownies bake efficiently in the Instant Vortex. Alternatively, one can reheat "last night's meal" for lunch, fresh as ever.

Design & Key Features

- Large capacity
- A basket that is large and square
- Easy-to-maintain and clean compartment

Instant vortex makes the crunchy food one would get from a traditional deep fryer by only adding a little oil to the food that's easily heated to cooking temperatures. This air fryer guarantees the foods are crispy on the exterior but juicy on the inside by air frying them easily and using only a small portion of the oil used in conventional frying or cooking. If one used to bake or cook the foods in the air fryer, they would notice that the results from an air fryer are much more scrumptious than those from a deep fryer, which can quickly dry out food that's fully cooked. Compared to the circle or round smaller buckets of most air fryers, the Vortex's square bowl is an important size difference; Instant Pot has enough space to cook a whole chicken. The Vortex's square design allows to use every inch of counter space to cram more food into the tray, which is big enough to serve a crowd.

Please notice this is a very bulky gadget (about 30cm wide and 32cm high). If one doesn't have enough space to keep it on the countertop, they will need to pack it away while not in use. The screen and dial are easy to use, with no awkward choices or over-complications. Before air-frying, the system sends out a signal until it's preheated. When it's time to rotate the food

– however, one can skip the latter if they are cooking for 1 to 2 individuals because smaller amounts of food cook even more evenly due to the circulating air therefore there is no need to rotate or flip the food at all.

Instant Vortex's Performance

- It is said that it uses up to 90% less oil than roasting and frying
- For packaged foods like potato waffles and air fryer chips, it's super-fast.
- Keeps leftovers crisp and juicy.

For a beautifully crispy feel, whole buckets of food just demanded a tbsp. of oil. Thankfully, the cooking tray drains extra oil, meaning the food doesn't sucks up any further after the cooking period is up.

As you know, cooking food in the air fryer takes a long time, as the opening of the door lets the hot air out and lengthens the entire cooking process. On the other hand, the air fryer requires less time and the heating environment is much more controlled. Many who are contemplating purchasing an air fryer, are concerned about the noise. Although the Vortex can create a whirring sound while operating, it is comparable to that of an extractor fan. Because cooking times seldom reach 20 to 30 minutes, it isn't anything that will deter anyone from having one. And, if the Vortex's multiple powers weren't enough, it also enables heating and frying a variety of processed foods: from arancini, spring rolls to popcorn, cheese toasties, and roti. It's great for foods that need very little oil but aren't wet from the outside. It made us realize how much oil is in popular foods like chips, potato waffles, etc. which all come out crisp and succulent after just a few minutes in the air fryer.

If the health advantages of consuming less oil aren't enough, one won't have to cope with the cooking scents that may persist for days after deep-frying meals, nor with any residual oil. If you have infants, is better to have The Vortex on the countertop than the normal fryer that uses hot oil.

Air Fryer Set Up Tips

Preheat your air fryer – this seems self-evident, but do not be like those who turn it on and then get upset when the fries aren't cooked (as mentioned in the recipe's) in 11 to 15-minute point. To cook something, it must first reach the proper temperature, much like the home air fryer. Alternatively, one might use the pressure cooker. It must first build up pressure before beginning to pressure cook.

Brush the pan or basket with oil – a thin brushing of oil would be enough to save the foods from sticking.

Do Not Directly Use Oil Spray– nonstick aerosol sprays will cause the air fryer to malfunction. Coat the tray and foods with an oil mister.

Cooking Tips with Air Frying

Oil Coating – Even if this is an instant vortex air fryer, one may also need to apply a little oil to assist with the "fry" portion. Lightly cover the food in oil before placing it in the air fryer. If one is cooking fat food like pork, there's no need to cover them in oil.

Keep it simple – never clutter the air fryer. Only certain items will crisp if you do this, while others will be damp or not browned.

Cook in batches to keep the single layer. This means that the meals are golden brown and crispy.

Flip it or shake it – To ensure even heating, take the basket out and shake every few minutes throughout the cooking phase. Remove the tray if you have one, rotate the food, and finish air frying.

Oil spray halfway through – If one wants everything to be very crispy, they should gently mist it with oil halfway through air frying. Only do this if the basket has been removed from the air fryer. If the basket is in the unit, do not apply the oil. If you add the oil to the machine while it's already running, it will create a messy build up and sludge inside.

Maintenance tips

Smoke: if in use, especially with oily foods like beef or bacon, the air fryer may emit white smoke. Don't be frightened. To stop this, add about two tablespoons of water to the bottom of the air fryer or a bread slice to the bottom of the air fryer to soak up some fat. Not only can the bread fix the smoke dilemma, but it will also help to trap the fat and the cleaning process after use will be easier

Preheating - Make sure to always preheat your air fryer. You will have long lasting performances

Washing – Wash the basket or tray with warm soapy water. If one has a metal plate, use a nylon Bristol cleaner to help clean out the tiny crevices.

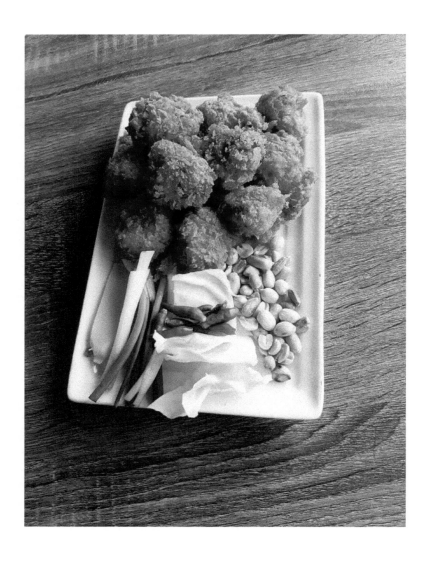

ALLSPICE CHICKEN WINGS

Preparation Time:| Cooking Time: 45 minutes | **Servings:** 8

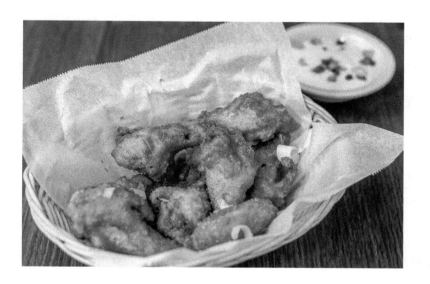

INGREDIENTS:

- ½ tsp celery salt

- ½ tsp bay leaf powder

- ½ tsp ground black pepper

- ½ tsp paprika

- ¼ tsp dry mustard

- ¼ tsp cayenne pepper

- ¼ tsp allspice

- 2 pounds chicken wings

DIRECTIONS:

1. Grease the air fryer basket and preheat to 340°F. In a bowl, mix celery salt, bay leaf powder, black pepper, paprika, dry mustard, cayenne pepper, and allspice.

2. Coat the wings thoroughly in this mixture.

3. Arrange the wings in an even layer in the basket of the air fryer. Cook the chicken until it's no longer pinks around the bone, for 30 minutes then, increase the temperature to 380°F and cook for 6 minutes more, until crispy on the outside.

NUTRITION:

Calories 332 | Fat 10.1 g | Carb 31.3 g | Protein 12 g

BALSAMIC ZUCCHINI SLICES

Preparation Time: 5 minutes | **Cooking Time:** 50 minutes | **Servings:** 6

INGREDIENTS:

- zucchinis, thinly sliced

- Salt and black pepper to taste

- tablespoons avocado oil

- tablespoons balsamic vinegar

DIRECTIONS:

1. Put all of the ingredients into a bowl and mix.

2. Put the zucchini mixture in your air fryer's basket and cook at 220°F for 50 minutes.

3. Serve as a snack and enjoy!

NUTRITION:

Calories 40 | Fat 3g | Fiber 7g | Carb 3g | Protein 7g

TURMERIC CARROT CHIPS

Preparation Time: 5 minutes | **Cooking Time:** 25 minutes | **Servings:** 4

INGREDIENTS:

- carrots, thinly sliced

- Salt and black pepper to taste

- ½ teaspoon turmeric powder

- ½ teaspoon chaat masala

- 1 teaspoon olive oil

DIRECTIONS:

1. Put all of the ingredients in a bowl and toss well.

2. Put the mixture in your air fryer's basket and cook at 370°F for 25 minutes, shaking the fryer from time to time.

3. Serve as a snack.

NUTRITION:

Calories 161 | Fat 1g | Fiber 2g | Carb 5g | Protein 3g

CRISP KALE

Preparation Time: 5 Minutes | **Cooking Time:** 8 Minutes | **Servings:** 2

INGREDIENTS:

- 4 Handfuls Kale, Washed & Stemless
- 1 Tablespoon Olive Oil
- Pinch Sea Salt

DIRECTIONS:

1. Start by heating it to 360°F, and then combine your ingredients together making sure your kale is coated evenly.

2. Place the kale in your fryer and cook for 8 minutes.

NUTRITION:

Calories 121 | Fat 4g | Carb 5g | Protein 8g

CHIVES RADISH SNACK

Preparation Time: 5 minutes | **Cooking Time:** 10 minutes | **Servings:** 4

INGREDIENTS:

- 16 radishes, sliced
- A drizzle of olive oil
- Salt and black pepper to taste
- 1 tablespoon chives, chopped

DIRECTIONS:

1. In a bowl, mix the radishes, salt, pepper, and oil; toss well.
2. Place the radishes in your air fryer's basket and cook at 350°F for 10 minutes.
3. Divide into bowls and serve with chives sprinkled on top.

NUTRITION:

Calories 100 | Fat 1g | Fiber 2g | Carb 4g | Protein 1g

Jicama Fries

Preparation Time: 10 minutes | **Cooking Time:** 5 minutes | **Servings:** 4

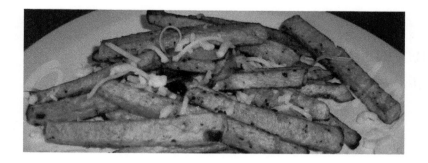

INGREDIENTS:

- 1 tbsp. dried thyme
- ¾ C. arrowroot flour
- ½ large Jicama
- eggs

DIRECTIONS:

1. Preparing the ingredients. Sliced jicama into fries.
2. Whisk eggs together and pour over fries. Toss to coat.

3. Mix a pinch of salt, thyme, and arrowroot flour together. Toss egg-coated jicama into dry mixture, tossing to coat well.

4. Air Frying. Spray the air fryer basket with olive oil and add fries. Set temperature to 350°F, and set time to 5 minutes. Toss halfway into the cooking process.

NUTRITION:

Calories 211 | Fat 19g | Carbs 16g | Protein 9g

Lentils Snack

Preparation Time: 5 Minutes | **Cooking Time:** 12 minutes | **Servings:** 4

INGREDIENTS:

- 15 ounces canned lentils, drained
- ½ teaspoon cumin, ground
- 1 tablespoon olive oil
- 1 teaspoon sweet paprika
- Salt and black pepper to taste

DIRECTIONS:

1. Place all ingredients in a bowl and blend it well.
2. Transfer the mixture to your air fryer and cook at 400°F for 12 minutes.
3. Divide into bowls and serve as a snack or a side, or appetizer!

NUTRITION:

Calories 151 | Fat 1g | Fiber 6g | Carb 10g | Protein 6g

CRUNCHY BACON BITES

Preparation Time: 5 minutes | **Cooking Time**: 5 minutes | **Servings:** 4

INGREDIENTS:

- bacon strips, cut into small pieces
- 1/2 cup pork rinds, crushed
- 1/4 cup hot sauce

DIRECTIONS:

1 Add bacon pieces in a bowl.
2 Add hot sauce and toss well.
3 Add crushed pork rinds and toss until bacon pieces are well coated.
4 Transfer bacon pieces in air fryer oven basket and cook at 350°F for 5minutes.
5 Serve and enjoy.

NUTRITION:

Calories 112 | Fat 9.7g | Carb 0.3g | Sugar 0.2g | Protein 5.2g

PESTO TOMATOES

Preparation Time: 5 minutes | **Cooking Time:** 10 minutes | **Servings:** 4

INGREDIENTS:

- Large heirloom tomatoes – 3, cut into ½ inch thick slices.

- Pesto – 1 cup

- Feta cheese – 8 oz. cut into ½ inch thick slices

- Red onion – ½ cup, sliced thinly

- Olive oil – 1 tbsp.

DIRECTIONS:

1. Spread some pesto on each slice of tomato. Top each tomato slice with a feta slice and onion and drizzle with oil. Arrange the tomatoes onto the greased rack and spray with cooking spray.

2. Preheat the Air Fryer to 390°F. Arrange the drip pan in the bottom of Air Fryer Oven cooking chamber and cook for 14 minutes.

3. Serve warm.

NUTRITION:

Calories 480 | Carb 13g | Fat 41.9g | Protein 15.4g

APPLE CHIPS

Preparation Time: 10 minutes | **Cooking Time:** 20 minutes | **Servings:** 2

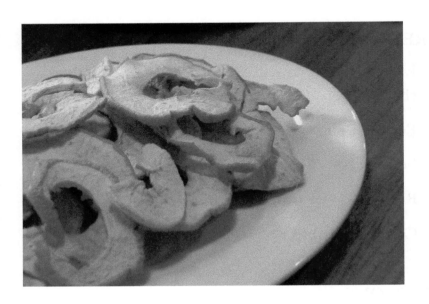

INGREDIENTS:

- 1 apple, sliced thinly

- Salt to taste

- ¼ teaspoon ground cinnamon

DIRECTIONS:

1. Preheat the air fryer to 350°F.

2. Toss the apple slices in salt and cinnamon.

3. Add to the air fryer.

4. Let cool before serving.

NUTRITION:

Calories 59 | Protein 0.3g | Fat 0.2g | Carb 15.6g

AIR FRIED HONEY ROASTED CARROTS

Preparation Time: 5 minutes | **Cooking Time:** 15 minutes | **Servings:** 4

INGREDIENTS:

- 3 cups baby carrots
- 1 tablespoon extra-virgin olive oil
- 1 tablespoon honey
- Salt
- Freshly ground black pepper
- Fresh dill (optional)

DIRECTIONS:

1. Preparing the ingredients. In a bowl, combine honey, olive oil, carrots, salt, and pepper. Make sure that the carrots are thoroughly coated with oil. Place the carrots in the air fryer basket.

2. Air Frying. Set the temperature to 390°F. Set the timer and roast for 12 minutes, or until fork-tender.

3. Remove the air fryer drawer and release the air fryer basket. Pour the carrots into a bowl, sprinkle with dill, if desired, and serve.

NUTRITION:

Calories 140 | Fat 3g | Carb 7g | Protein 9g

FRENCH TOAST STICKS

Preparation Time: 5 minutes | **Cooking Time:** 15 minutes | **Servings:** 12

INGREDIENTS:

- 4 slices Texas toast (or any thick bread, such as challah)
- 1 tablespoon butter
- 1 egg
- 1 teaspoon stevia
- 1 teaspoon ground cinnamon
- ¼ cup milk
- 1 teaspoon vanilla extract
- Cooking oil

DIRECTIONS:

1. Cut each slice of bread into 3 pieces (for 12 sticks total).

2. Place the butter in a small, microwave-safe bowl. Heat for 15 seconds, or until the butter has melted.

3. Remove the bowl from the microwave. Add the egg, stevia, cinnamon, milk, and vanilla extract. Whisk until fully combined.

4. Sprinkle the air fryer with cooking oil.

5. Dredge each of the bread sticks in the egg mixture.

6. Place the French toast sticks in the air fryer. It is okay to stack them. Spray the French toast sticks with cooking oil. Cook for 8 minutes

7. Open the air fryer and flip each of the French toast sticks. Cook for an additional 4 minutes, or until the French toast sticks are crisp.

8. Cool before serving.

NUTRITION:

Calories 52 | Fat 2g | Carb 7g | Protein 2g

Pepperoni Chips

Preparation Time: 2 minutes | Cooking Time: 5 minutes | Servings: 6

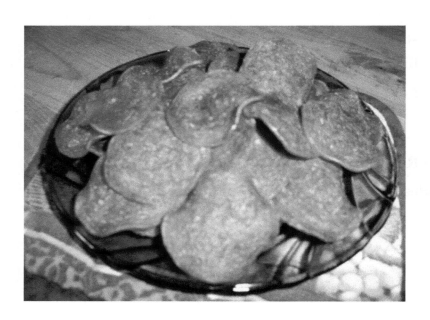

INGREDIENTS :

- oz pepperoni slices

DIRECTIONS:

1 Place one batch of pepperoni slices in the air fryer oven basket.
2 Cook for 5 minutes at 360°F.
3 Cook remaining pepperoni slices using same steps.

4   Serve and enjoy.

NUTRITION:

Calories 51 | Fat 1g | Carb 2g | Sugar 1.3g | Protein 0g

MUSHROOM PITA PIZZAS

Preparation Time: 5 minutes | Cooking Time: 5 minutes | Servings: 4

INGREDIENTS:

- (3-inch) pitas
- 1 tablespoon olive oil
- ¾ cup pizza sauce
- 1 (4-ounce) jar sliced mushrooms, drained
- ½ teaspoon dried basil
- green onions, minced
- 1 cup grated mozzarella or provolone cheese
- 1 cup sliced grape tomatoes

DIRECTIONS:

1   Brush each piece of pita with oil and top with the pizza sauce.

2   Add the mushrooms and sprinkle with basil and green onions. Top with the grated cheese.

3   Bake for 5 minutes or until the cheese is melted and starts to brown. Top with the grape tomatoes and serve immediately.

42

NUTRITION:

Calories 231| Fat 9g | Carb 25g| Fiber 2g | Protein 13g

SHRIMP AND GRILLED CHEESE SANDWICHES

Preparation Time: 5 minutes | **Cooking Time**: 5 minutes | **Servings**: 4

INGREDIENTS:

- 1¼ cups shredded Colby, Cheddar, or Havarti cheese
- 1 (6-ounce) can tiny shrimp, drained
- tablespoons mayonnaise
- tablespoons minced green onion
- slices whole grain or whole-wheat bread
- tablespoons softened butt

DIRECTIONS:

1. In a medium bowl, combine the cheese, shrimp, mayonnaise, and green onion, and mix well.

2. Spread this mixture on two of the slices of bread. Top with the other slices of bread to make two sandwiches. Spread the sandwiches lightly with butter.

3. Grill in the air fryer for 5 to 7 minutes or until the bread is browned and crisp and the cheese is melted. Cut in half and serve warm.

NUTRITION:

Calories 276 | Fat 14g | Carb 16g | Fiber 2g | Protein 22g

BURRATA-STUFFED TOMATOES

Preparation Time: 5 minutes | **Cooking Time:** 5 minutes | **Servings:** 4

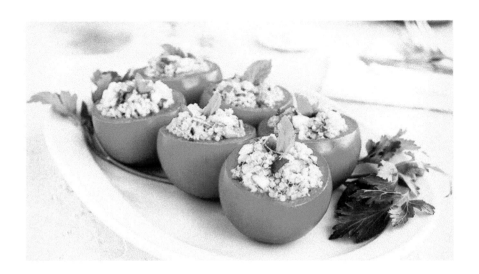

INGREDIENTS:

- 4 medium tomatoes

- ½ teaspoon fine sea salt

- 4 (2-ounce) Burrata balls

- Fresh basil leaves, for garnish

- Extra-virgin olive oil, for drizzling

DIRECTIONS:

1. Preparing the ingredients. Preheat the air fryer to 300°F.

2. Scoop out the tomato seeds and membranes using a melon baller or spoon. Sprinkle the insides of the tomatoes with the salt. Stuff each tomato with a ball of Burrata.

3. Air Frying. Put it in the fryer and cook for 5 minutes, or until the cheese has softened.

4. Garnish with olive oil and basil leaves. Serve warm.

NUTRITION:

Calories 108 | Fat 7g | Protein 6g | Total Carb 5g | Fiber 2g

FLATBREAD

Preparation Time: 5 minutes | **Cooking Time:** 5 minutes | **Servings:** 2

INGREDIENTS:

- 1 cup shredded mozzarella cheese

- ¼ cup almond flour

- 1-ounce full-fat cream cheese softened

DIRECTIONS:

1. Melt mozzarella in the microwave for 30 seconds. Stir in almond flour until smooth.

2. Add cream cheese. Continue mixing until dough forms. Knead with wet hands if necessary.

3. Divide the dough into two pieces and roll out to ¼-inch thickness between two pieces of parchment.

4. Cover the air fryer basket with parchment and place the flatbreads into the air fryer basket. Work in batches if necessary.

5. Cook at 320°F for 5 minutes. Flip once at the halfway mark.

6. Serve.

NUTRITION:

Calories 296 | Fat 22.6g | Carb 3.3g | Protein 16.3g

VEGETABLE EGG ROLLS

Preparation Time: 5 minutes | **Cooking Time:** 5 minutes | **Servings:** 8

INGREDIENTS:

- ½ cup chopped mushrooms

- ½ cup grated carrots

- ½ cup chopped zucchini

- green onions, chopped

- tablespoons low-sodium soy sauce

- egg roll wrappers

- 1 tablespoon cornstarch

- 1 egg, beaten

DIRECTIONS:

1   In a medium bowl, combine the mushrooms, carrots, zucchini, green onions, and soy sauce, and stir together.

2   Place the egg roll wrappers on a work surface. Top each with about 3 tablespoons of the vegetable mixture.

3   In a small bowl, combine the cornstarch and egg and mix well. Brush some of this mixture on the edges of the egg roll wrappers. Roll up the wrappers, enclosing the vegetable filling. Brush some of the egg mixture on the outside of the egg rolls to seal.

4   Air-fry for 5 minutes or until the egg rolls are brown and crunchy.

NUTRITION:

Calories 112| Fat 1g | Carb 21g| Fiber 1g | Protein 4g

SPINACH FRITTATA

Preparation Time: 5 minutes | **Cooking Time:** 8 minutes | **Servings:** 1

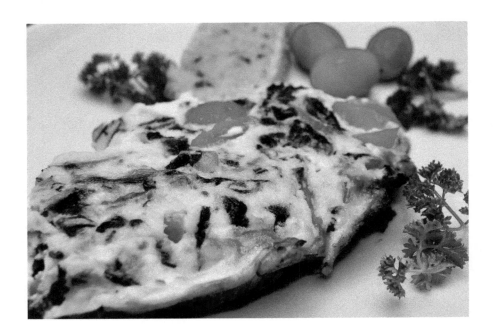

INGREDIENTS:

- 3 eggs
- 1 cup spinach, chopped
- 1 small onion, minced
- 2 tbsp mozzarella cheese, grated
- Pepper

- Salt

DIRECTIONS:

1. Preheat the air fryer to 350°F. Spray air fryer pan with cooking spray.

2. In a bowl, whisk eggs with remaining ingredients until well combined.

3. Pour egg mixture into the prepared pan and place pan in the air fryer.

4. Cook frittata for 8 minutes or until set. Serve and enjoy.

NUTRITION:

Calories 384 | Fat 23.3 g | Carb 10.7 g | Protein 34.3 g

TUNA ZUCCHINI MELTS

Preparation Time: 15 minutes | **Cooking Time**: 5 minutes | **Servings:** 4

INGREDIENTS:

- corn tortillas

- tablespoons softened butter

- 1 (6-ounce) can chunk light tuna, drained

- 1 cup shredded zucchini, drained by squeezing in a kitchen towel

- ⅓ cup mayonnaise

- tablespoons mustard

- 1 cup shredded Cheddar or Colby cheese

DIRECTIONS:

1. Spread the tortillas with the softened butter. Place in the air fryer basket and grill for 2 to 3 minutes or until the tortillas are crisp. Remove from basket and set aside.

2. In a medium bowl, combine the tuna, zucchini, mayonnaise, and mustard, and mix well.

3. Divide the tuna mixture among the toasted tortillas. Top each with some of the shredded cheese.

4. Grill in the air fryer for 2 to 4 minutes or until the tuna mixture is hot, and the cheese melts and starts to brown. Serve.

NUTRITION:

Calories 428 | Fat 30g | Carb 19g | Fiber 3g | Protein 22g

BREADED MUSHROOMS

Preparation Time: 10 minutes | **Cooking Time:** 45 minutes | **Servings:** 4

INGREDIENTS:

- 1 lb. small Button mushrooms, cleaned
- cups breadcrumbs
- eggs, beaten
- Salt and pepper to taste
- 2 cups Parmigiano Reggiano cheese, grated

DIRECTIONS:

1. Preheat the Air Fryer to 360°F. Pour the breadcrumbs in a bowl, add salt and pepper and mix well. Pour the cheese in a separate bowl and set aside. Dip each mushroom in the eggs, then in the crumbs, and then in the cheese.

2. Slide out the fryer basket and add 6 to 10 mushrooms. Cook them for 20 minutes, in batches, if needed. Serve with cheese dip.

NUTRITION:

Calories 487 | Carb 49g | Fat 22g | Protein 31g

Bacon Wrapped Avocados

Preparation Time: 10 minutes | **Cooking Time:** 30 minutes | **Servings:** 4

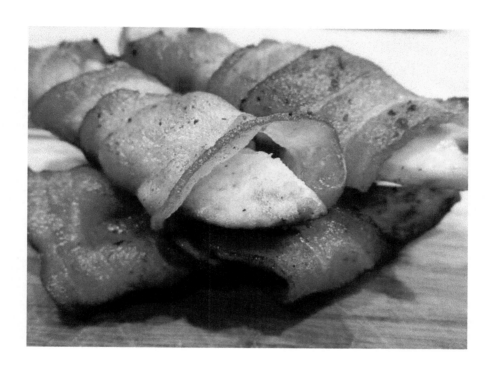

INGREDIENTS:

- 12 thick strips bacon

- large avocados, sliced

- ⅓ tsp salt

- ⅓ tsp chili powder

- ⅓ tsp cumin powder

DIRECTIONS:

1 Stretch the bacon strips to elongate and use a knife to cut in half to make 24 pieces. Wrap each bacon piece around a slice of avocado from one end to the other end.

2 Tuck the end of bacon into the wrap. Arrange on a flat surface and season with salt, chili and cumin on both sides.

3 Arrange 4 to 8 wrapped pieces in the air fryer and cook at 350°F for 8 minutes, or until the bacon is browned and crunchy, flipping halfway through to cook evenly. Remove onto a wire rack and repeat the process for the remaining avocado pieces.

NUTRITION:

Calories 193 | Carb 10g | Fat 16g | Protein 4g

Cheesy Sticks with Sweet Thai Sauce

Preparation Time: 2 hours | **Cooking Time:** 20 minutes | **Servings:** 4

INGREDIENTS:

- 12 mozzarella string cheese
- cups breadcrumbs
- eggs
- 1 cup sweet Thai sauce
- tbsp skimmed milk

DIRECTIONS:

1. Pour the crumbs in a medium bowl. Break the eggs into a different bowl and beat with the milk. One after the other, dip each cheese sticks in the egg mixture, in the crumbs, then egg mixture again and then in the crumbs again.

2. Place the coated cheese sticks on a cookie sheet and freeze for 1 to 2 hours. Preheat the Air Fryer to 380°F. Arrange the sticks in the fryer without overcrowding. Cook for 5 minutes, flipping them

halfway through cooking to brown evenly. Cook in batches. Serve with a sweet Thai sauce.

NUTRITION:

Calories 158 | Carb 14g | Fat 7g | Protein 9g

CRISPY BRUSSELS SPROUTS

Preparation Time: 5 minutes | **Cooking Time:** 10 minutes | **Servings:** 2

INGREDIENTS:

- ½ pound brussels sprouts, cut in half

- ½ tablespoon oil

- ½ tablespoon unsalted butter, melted

DIRECTIONS:

3. Rub sprouts with oil and place into the air fryer basket.

4. Cook at 400°F for 10 minutes. Stir once at the halfway mark.

5. Remove the air fryer basket and drizzle with melted butter.

6. Serve.

NUTRITION:

Calories 90 | Fat 6.1g | Carb 4g | Protein 2.9g

ROASTED ALMONDS

Preparation Time: 5 minutes | Cooking Time:5 minutes | Servings: 8

INGREDIENTS:

- cups almonds
- 1/4 tsp pepper
- 1 tsp paprika
- 1 tbsp garlic powder
- 1 tbsp soy sauce

DIRECTIONS:

1   Add pepper, paprika, garlic powder, and soy sauce in a bowl and stir well.
2   Add almonds and stir to coat.
3   Spray air fryer oven basket with cooking spray.
4   Add almonds in air fryer oven basket and cook for 5 minutes at 320°F..
5   Serve and enjoy.

NUTRITION:

Calories 143 | Fat 11.9 g | Carb 6.2 g | Sugar 1.3 g | Protein 5.4 g

SIMPLE GARLIC POTATOES

Preparation Time: 5Minutes | **Cooking Time:** 5 Minutes | **Servings:** 2

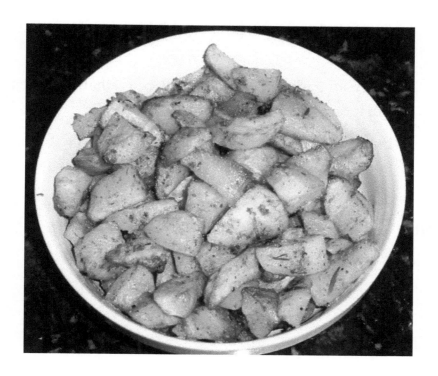

INGREDIENTS:

- 3 Baking Potatoes, Large
- 2 Tablespoons Olive Oil
- 2 Tablespoons Garlic, Minced
- 1 Tablespoon Salt

- ½ Tablespoon Onion Powder

DIRECTIONS:

1. Turn on your air fryer to 390°F.

2. Create holes in your potato, and then sprinkle it with oil and salt.

3. Mix your garlic and onion powder together, and then rub it on the potatoes evenly.

4. Put it into your air fryer basket, and then bake for 5 minutes.

NUTRITION:

Calories 160 | Fat 6g | Carb 9g | Protein 9g

ZUCCHINI CUBES

Preparation Time: 5 minutes | **Cooking Time:** 5 minutes | **Servings:** 2

INGREDIENTS:

- 1 zucchini
- ½ teaspoon ground black pepper
- 1 teaspoon oregano
- 2 tablespoons chicken stock
- ½ teaspoon coconut oil

DIRECTIONS:

1. Chop the zucchini into cubes.

2. Combine the ground black pepper, and oregano; stir the mixture.

3. Sprinkle the zucchini cubes with the spice mixture and stir well.

4. After this, sprinkle the vegetables with the chicken stock.

5. Place the coconut oil in the air fryer basket and preheat it to 360°F for 20 seconds.

6. Then add the zucchini cubes and cook the vegetables for 5 minutes at 390°F, stirring halfway through.

7. Transfer to serving plates and enjoy!

NUTRITION:

Calories 30 | Fat 1.5g | Fiber 1.6g | Carb 4.3g | Protein 1.4g

CARROT CRISPS

Preparation Time: 10 minutes | **Cooking Time:** 10 minutes | **Servings:** 4

INGREDIENTS:

- large carrots, washed and peeled
- Salt to taste
- Cooking spray

DIRECTIONS:

1   Using a mandolin slicer, slice the carrots very thinly height wise. Put the carrot strips in a bowl and season with salt to taste.

2   Grease the fryer basket lightly with cooking spray, and add the carrot strips.

3   Cook at 350°F for 10 minutes, stirring once halfway through.

NUTRITION:

Calories 35 | Carb 8g | Fat 3g | Protein 1g

Quick Cheese Sticks

Preparation Time: 5 minutes | **Cooking Time:** 10 minutes | **Servings:** 4

INGREDIENTS:

- 6 oz bread cheese
- tbsp butter
- cups panko crumbs

DIRECTIONS:

1   Place the butter in a dish and melt it in the microwave, for 2 minutes; set aside. With a knife, cut the cheese into equal sized sticks.

2   Brush each stick with butter and dip into panko crumbs. Arrange the cheese sticks in a single layer on the fryer basket.

3   Cook at 390°F for 10 minutes. Flip them halfway through, to brown evenly; serve warm.

NUTRITION:

Calories 256 | Carb 8g | Fat 21g | Protein 16g

HOT CHICKEN WINGETTES

Preparation Time: 10 minutes | **Cooking Time:** 40 minutes | **Servings:** 4

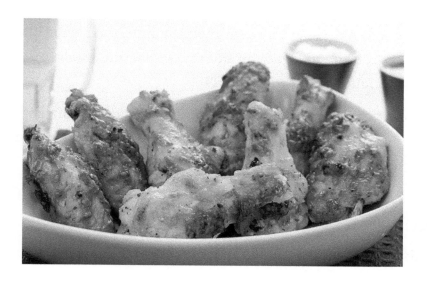

INGREDIENTS:

- 15 chicken wingettes
- Salt and pepper to taste
- ⅓ cup hot sauce
- ⅓ cup butter
- ½ tbsp vinegar

DIRECTIONS:

1   Preheat the Air Fryer to 360°F. Season the vignettes with pepper and salt. Add them to the air fryer and cook for 35 minutes.

2   Toss every 5 minutes. Once ready, remove them into a bowl. Over low heat melt the butter in a saucepan. Add the vinegar and hot sauce. Stir and cook for a minute.

3   Turn the heat off. Pour the sauce over the chicken. Toss to coat well. Transfer the chicken to a serving platter. Serve with blue cheese dressing.

NUTRITION:

Calories 563 | Carb 2g | Fat 28g | Protein 35g

Radish Chips

Preparation Time: 10 minutes | **Cooking Time:** 20 minutes | **Servings:** 4

INGREDIENTS:

- radishes, leaves removed and cleaned

- Salt to season

- Water

- Cooking spray

DIRECTIONS:

1   Using a mandolin, slice the radishes thinly. Put them in a pot and pour water on them. Heat the pot on a stovetop, and bring to boil, until the radishes are translucent, for 4 minutes. After 4 minutes, drain the radishes through a sieve; set aside. Grease the fryer basket with cooking spray.

2   Add in the radish slices and cook for 8 minutes, flipping once halfway through. Cook until golden brown, at 400°F. Meanwhile, prepare a paper towel-lined plate. Once the radishes are ready, transfer them to the paper towel-lined plate. Season with salt, and serve with ketchup or garlic mayo.

NUTRITION:

Calories 25 | Carb 0.2g | Fat 2g | Protein 0.1g

HERBED CROUTONS WITH BRIE CHEESE

Preparation Time: 10 minutes | **Cooking Time:** 10 minutes | **Servings:** 4

INGREDIENTS:

- tbsp olive oil
- 1 tbsp french herbs
- oz brie cheese, chopped
- slices bread, halved

DIRECTIONS:

1 Warm up your Air Fryer to 340° F. Using a bowl, mix oil with herbs. Dip the bread slices in the oil mixture to coat.

2 Place the coated slices on a flat surface. Lay the brie cheese on the slices.

3 Place the slices into your air fryer's basket and cook for 7 minutes.

4 Once the bread is ready, cut into cubes.

NUTRITION:

Calories 20 | Carb 1.5g | Fat 1.3g | Protein 0.5g

ASPARAGUS FRITTATA

Preparation Time: 10 minutes | **Cooking Time:** 10 minutes | **Servings:** 4

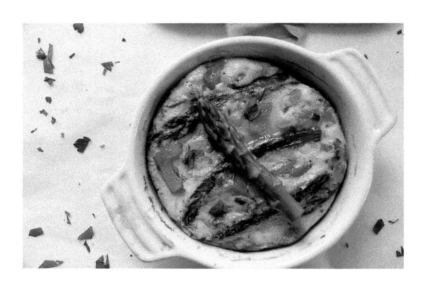

INGREDIENTS:

- 6 eggs

- 3 mushrooms, sliced

- 10 asparagus, chopped

- 1/4 cup half and half

- 2 tsp butter, melted

- 1 cup mozzarella cheese, shredded

- 1 tsp pepper

- 1 tsp salt

DIRECTIONS:

1. Toss mushrooms and asparagus with melted butter and add into the air fryer. Cook mushrooms and asparagus at 350°F for 5 minutes.

2. Meanwhile, in a bowl, whisk together eggs, half and half, pepper, and salt. Transfer cook mushrooms and asparagus into a proper dish. Pour egg mixture over mushrooms and asparagus.

3. Place dish in the air fryer and cook at 350°F for 5 minutes or until eggs are set. Slice and serve.

NUTRITION:

Calories 211 | Fat 13 g | Carb 4 g | Protein 16 g

CHIA SEED CRACKERS

Preparation Time: 15 minutes | **Cooking Time:** 45 minutes | **Servings:** 48

INGREDIENTS:

- 1 Cup raw chia seed
- 3/4 Teaspoon salt
- 1/4 Teaspoon garlic powder
- 1/4 Teaspoon onion powder
- 1 Cup cold water

DIRECTIONS:

1   Put the chia seeds in a bowl. Add salt, garlic powder, and onion powder.

2   Pour into the water. Stir. Cover with plastic wrap. Store in the fridge overnight. Preheat the Air fryer toaster oven to 200°F. Cover a baking sheet with a silicone mat or parchment. Transfer the soaked linseed to a prepared baking sheet.

3   Scatter it out with a spatula in a thin, flat rectangle about 1 cm thick. Rate the rectangle in about 32 small rectangles.

4   Bake in the preheated Air fryer toaster oven up to the chia seeds have darkened and contract slightly, about 3 hours. Let it cool. Break individual cookies.

NUTRITION:

Calories 120 | Fat 3.9 g | Carb 1.9 g | Protein 1.9g

FLAX SEED CHIPS

Preparation Time: 5 minutes | **Cooking Time:** 15 minutes | **Servings:** 4

INGREDIENTS:

- 1 Cup almond flour
- 1/2 Cup flax seeds
- 1 1/2 Teaspoons seasoned salt
- 1 Teaspoon sea salt
- 1/2 Cup water

DIRECTIONS:

1   Preheat the Air fryer toaster oven to 340°F.

2   Combine almond flour, flax seeds, 1 1/2 teaspoons seasoned salt and sea salt in a container; Stir in the water up to the dough is completely mixed. Shape the dough into narrow size slices the size of a bite and place them on a baking sheet. Sprinkle the rounds with seasoned salt.

3   Bake in preheated air fryer toaster oven up to crispy, about 15 minutes.

4   Cool fully and store in an airtight box or in a sealed bag.

NUTRITION:

Calories 126.9 | Fat 6.1g | Carb 15.9 g | Protein 2.9g

Stuffed Jalapeno

Preparation Time: 10 minutes | **Cooking Time:** 10 minutes | **Servings:** 4

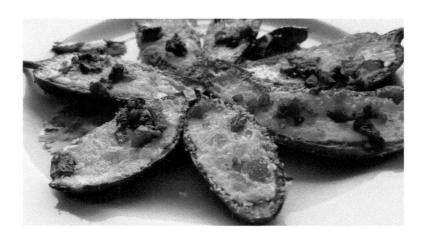

INGREDIENTS:

- 1 lb. ground pork sausage

- 1 (8 oz.) package cream cheese, softened

- 1 cup shredded Parmesan cheese

- 1 lb. large fresh jalapeno peppers halved lengthwise and seeded

- 1 (8 oz.) bottle Ranch dressing

DIRECTIONS:

1   in Mix pork sausage ground with ranch dressing and cream cheese in a bowl. But the jalapeno in half and remove their seeds.

2   Divide the cream cheese mixture into the jalapeno halves.

3   Place the jalapeno pepper in a baking tray. Set the Baking tray inside the Air Fryer toaster oven and close the lid. Select the Bake mode at 350°F for 10 minutes.

4   Serve warm.

NUTRITION:

Calories 168| Protein 9.4g | Carb 12.1g | Fat 21.2g

Salted Hazelnuts

Preparation Time: 15 minutes | **Cooking Time:** 10 minutes | **Servings:** 8

INGREDIENTS:

- Cups dry roasted Hazelnuts, no salt added
- Tablespoons coconut oil
- 1 Teaspoon garlic powder
- 1 Sprig fresh Thyme, chopped
- 1 1/2 Teaspoons salt

DIRECTIONS:

1   Preheat the Air fryer toaster oven to 350°F.

2   Mix the Hazelnuts, coconut oil, garlic powder and thyme in a bowl until the nuts are fully covered.

3   Sprinkle with salt. Spread evenly on a baking sheet.

4   Bake in the preheated Air fryer toaster oven for 10 minutes.

NUTRITION:

Calories 237 | Fat 21.3 g | Carb 5.9 g | Protein 7.4g

CAJUN OLIVES AND PEPPERS

Preparation Time: 4 minutes | **Cooking Time:** 12 minutes | **Servings:** 4

INGREDIENTS:

- 1 tablespoon olive oil

- ½ pound mixed bell peppers, sliced

- 1 cup black olives, pitted and halved

- ½ tablespoon Cajun seasoning

DIRECTIONS:

1. In a pan that fits the air fryer, combine all the ingredients.

2. Put the pan it in your air fryer and cook at 390°F for 12 minutes.

3. Divide the mix between plates and serve.

NUTRITION:

Calories 151 | Fat 3g | Fiber 2g | Carb 4g | Protein 5g

YOGURT BREAD

Preparation Time: 20 minutes | **Cooking Time:** 40 minutes | **Servings:** 10

INGREDIENTS:

- 1½ cups warm water, divided
- 1½ teaspoons active dry yeast
- 1 teaspoon sugar
- 3 cups all-purpose flour
- 1 cup plain Greek yogurt
- 2 teaspoons kosher salt

DIRECTIONS:

1. Add ½ cup of the warm water, yeast and sugar in the bowl of a stand mixer, fitted with the dough hook attachment and mix well.

2. Set aside for about 5 minutes

3. Add the flour, yogurt, and salt and mix on medium-low speed until the dough comes together.

4. Then, mix on medium speed for 5 minutes

5. Place the dough into a bowl.

6. With a plastic wrap, cover the bowl and place in a warm place for about 2-3 hours or until doubled in size.

7. Transfer the dough onto a lightly floured surface and shape into a smooth ball.

8. Place the dough onto a greased parchment paper-lined rack.

9. With a kitchen towel, cover the dough and let rest for 15 minutes

10. With a very sharp knife, cut a 4x½-inch deep cut down the center of the dough.

11. Take to the preheated air fryer at 325°F for 40 minutes.

12. Carefully, invert the bread to cool completely before slicing.

13. Cut the bread into desired-sized slices and serve.

NUTRITION:

Calories 157 | Fat 0.7 g | Carb 31 g | Protein 5.5 g

BACON-WRAPPED ASPARAGUS

Preparation Time: 5 minutes | **Cooking Time:** 10 minutes | **Servings:** 4

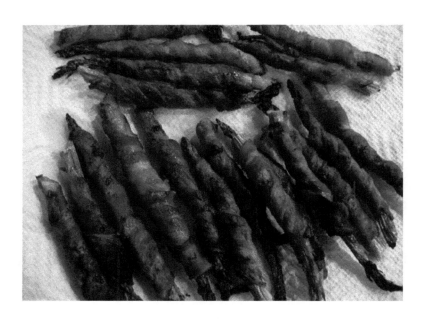

INGREDIENTS:

- 1 pound asparagus, trimmed (about 24 spears)

- 4slices bacon or beef bacon

- ½ cup Ranch Dressin for serving

- 3 tablespoons chopped fresh chives, for garnish

DIRECTIONS:

1. Preparing the ingredients. Grease the air fryer basket with avocado oil. Preheat the air fryer to 400°F.

2. Slice the bacon down the middle, making long, thin strips. Wrap 1 slice of bacon around 3 asparagus spears and secure each end with a toothpick. Repeat with the remaining bacon and asparagus.

3. Air Frying. Place the asparagus bundles in the air fryer in a single layer. (If you're using a smaller air fryer, cook in batches if necessary.) Cook for 8 minutes for thin stalks, 10 minutes for medium to thick stalks, or until the asparagus is slightly charred on the ends and the bacon is crispy.

4. Serve with ranch dressing and garnish with chives. Best served fresh.

NUTRITION:

Calories 241 | Fat 22g | Protein 7g | Carbs 6g | Fiber 3g

WRAPPED ASPARAGUS

Preparation Time: 10 minutes | **Cooking Time:** 5 minutes | **Servings:** 4

INGREDIENTS:

- 12 ounces asparagus
- ½ teaspoon ground black pepper
- 3-ounce turkey fillet, sliced
- ¼ teaspoon chili flakes

DIRECTIONS:

1. Sprinkle the asparagus with the ground black pepper and chili flakes.
2. Stir carefully.
3. Wrap the asparagus in the sliced turkey fillet and place in the air fryer basket.
4. Cook the asparagus at 400° F for 5 minutes, turning halfway through cooking.
5. Let the wrapped asparagus cool for 2 minutes before serving.

NUTRITION:

Calories 133 | Fat 9g | Fiber 1.9g | Carbs 3.8g | Protein 9.8g

GARLICKY BOK CHOY

Preparation Time: 10 minutes | **Cooking Time:** 10 minutes | **Servings:** 2

INGREDIENTS:

- bunches baby bok choy
- spray oil
- 1 tsp garlic powder

DIRECTIONS:

1 Toss bok choy with garlic powder and spread them in the Air fryer. Spray them with cooking oil.

2 Select the Air Fry mode at 350°F temperature for 6 minutes.

3 Serve fresh.

NUTRITION:

Calories 81 | Protein 0.4g | Carb 4.7g | Fat 8.3g

CHILI CORN ON THE COB

Preparation Time: 10 minutes | **Cooking Time:** 15 minutes | **Servings:** 4

INGREDIENTS:

- 2tablespoon olive oil, divided
- 2 tablespoons grated Parmesan cheese
- 1 teaspoon garlic powder
- 1 teaspoon chili powder
- 1 teaspoon ground cumin
- 1 teaspoon paprika
- 1 teaspoon salt
- ¼ teaspoon cayenne pepper (optional)
- 4ears fresh corn, shucked

DIRECTIONS:

1. Grease the air fryer basket with 1 tablespoon of olive oil. Set aside.

2. Combine the Parmesan cheese, garlic powder, chili powder, cumin, paprika, salt, and cayenne pepper (if desired) in a small bowl and stir to mix well.

3. Lightly coat the ears of corn with the remaining 1 tablespoon of olive oil. Rub the cheese mixture all over the ears of corn until completely coated.

4. Arrange the ears of corn in the greased basket in a single layer.

5. Put in the air fryer basket and cook at 400°F for 15 minutes.

6. Flip the ears of corn halfway through the cooking time.

7. When cooking is complete, they should be lightly browned. Remove from the oven and let them cool for 5 minutes before serving.

NUTRITION:

Calories 172 | Fat 9.8g | Carb 17.5g | Protein 3.9g

GREEN BEANS & BACON

Preparation Time: 15 minutes | **Cooking Time:** 20 minutes | **Servings:** 4

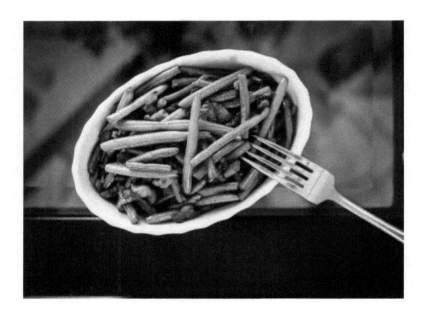

INGREDIENTS:

- 3 cups frozen cut green beans

- 1 medium onion, chopped

- 3 slices bacon, chopped

- ¼ cup water

- Kosher salt and black pepper

DIRECTIONS:

1. Preparing the ingredients. In a 6 × 3-inch round heatproof pan, combine the frozen green beans, onion, bacon, and water. Toss to combine. Place the saucepan in the basket.

2. Set the air fryer to 375°F for 15 minutes.

3. Raise the air fryer temperature to 400°F for 5 minutes. Season the beans with salt and pepper to taste and toss well.

4. Remove the pan from the air fryer basket and cover with foil.

5. Let it rest for 5 minutes then serve.

NUTRITION:

Calories 230 | Fat 10g | Carb 14g | Protein 17g

SIMPLE STUFFED POTATOES

Preparation Time: 15 Minutes | **Cooking Time:** 35 Minutes | **Servings:** 4

INGREDIENTS:

- 4 Large Potatoes, Peeled
- 2 Bacon, Rashers
- ½ Brown Onion, Diced
- ¼ Cup Cheese, Grated

DIRECTIONS:

1. Start by heating your air fryer to 350°F.

2. Cut your potatoes in half, and then brush the potatoes with oil.

3. Put it in your air fryer, and cook for ten minutes. Brush the potatoes with oil again and bake for another ten minutes.

4. Make a whole in the baked potato to get them ready to stuff.

5. Sauté the bacon and onion in a frying pan. You should do this over medium heat, adding cheese and stir. Remove from heat.

6. Stuff your potatoes, and cook for four to five minutes.

NUTRITION:

Calories 180 | Fat 8g | Carb 10g | Protein 11g

Ravishing Carrots with Honey Glaze

Preparation Time: 5 minutes | **Cooking Time:** 11 minutes | **Servings:** 1

INGREDIENTS:

- 3 cups of chopped into ½-inch pieces carrots
- 1 tablespoon of olive oil
- 2 tablespoons of honey
- 1 tablespoon of brown sugar
- salt and black pepper

DIRECTIONS:

1. Heat up your air fryer to 390°F.
2. Using a bowl, add and toss the carrot pieces, olive oil, honey, brown sugar, salt, and the black pepper until it is properly covered.
3. Place it inside your air fryer and add the seasoned glazed carrots.
4. Cook it for 5 minutes at 390°F, and then shake after 6 minutes. Serve and enjoy!

NUTRITION:

Calories 90 | Fat 3.5g | Fiber 2g | Carb 13g | Protein 1g

Omelet Frittata

Preparation Time: 10 minutes | **Cooking Time:** 6 minutes | **Servings:** 2

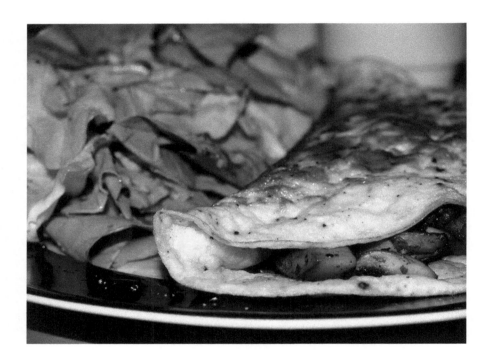

INGREDIENTS:

- 3 eggs, lightly beaten
- 2 tbsp cheddar cheese, shredded
- 2 tbsp heavy cream
- 2 mushrooms, sliced
- 1/4 small onion, chopped

- 1/4 bell pepper, diced
- Pepper
- Salt

DIRECTIONS:

1. In a bowl, whisk eggs with cream, vegetables, pepper, and salt.
2. Preheat the air fryer to 400°F.
3. Pour egg mixture into the air fryer pan. Place pan in air fryer and cook for 5 minutes
4. Add shredded cheese on top of the frittata and cook for 1 minute more.
5. Serve and enjoy.

NUTRITION:

Calories 160 | Fat 10 g | Carb 4 g | Protein 12 g

VEGGIES ON TOAST

Preparation Time: 12 minutes | **Cooking Time**: 10 minutes | **Servings:** 4

INGREDIENTS:

- 1 red bell pepper, cut into ½-inch strips
- 1 cup sliced button or cremini mushrooms
- 1 small yellow squash, sliced
- green onions, cut into ½-inch slices
- Extra light olive oil for misting
- to 6 pieces sliced French or Italian bread
- tablespoons softened butter
- ½ cup soft goat cheese

DIRECTIONS:

1. Combine the red pepper, mushrooms, squash, and green onions in the air fryer and mist with oil. Roast for 5 to 9 minutes or until the vegetables are tender, shaking the basket once during cooking time.

2. Remove the vegetables from the basket and set aside.

3. Spread the bread with butter and place in the air fryer, butter-side up. Toast for 2 to 4 minutes or until golden brown.

4. Spread the goat cheese on the toasted bread and top with the vegetables; serve warm.

5. Variation tip: To add even more flavor, drizzle the finished toasts with extra-virgin olive oil and balsamic vinegar.

NUTRITION:

Calories 162 | Fat 11g | Carb 9g | Fiber 2g | Protein 7g

FRIED PLANTAINS

Preparation Time: 5 minutes | **Cooking Time:** 10 minutes | **Servings:** 2

INGREDIENTS:

- 2ripe plantains, peeled and cut at a diagonal into ½-inch-thick pieces

- 3 tablespoons ghee, melted

- ¼ teaspoon kosher salt

DIRECTIONS:

1. Preparing the ingredients. In a bowl, mix the plantains with the ghee and salt.

2. Air Frying. Arrange the plantain pieces in the air fryer basket. Set the air fryer to 400°F for 8 minutes.

3. The plantains are done when they are soft and tender on the inside, and have plenty of crisp, sweet, brown spots on the outside.

NUTRITION:

Calories 180 | Fat 5g | Carb 10g | Protein 7g

SWEET POTATO FRIES

Preparation Time: 10 Minutes | **Cooking Time:** 12 Minutes | **Servings:** 2

INGREDIENTS:

- 3 Large Sweet Potatoes, Peeled
- 1 Tablespoon Olive Oil
- A Pinch Teaspoon Sea Salt

DIRECTIONS:

1. Turn on your air fryer to 390°F.

2. Start by cutting your sweet potatoes in quarters, cutting them lengthwise to make fries.

3. Combine the uncooked fries with a tablespoon of sea salt and olive oil. Make sure all of your fries are coated well.

4. Place your sweet potato pieces in your air fryer, cooking for 12 minutes.

5. Cook for two to three minutes more if you want it to be crispier.

6. Add more salt to taste, and serve when cooled.

NUTRITION:

Calories: 150 | Fat: 6g | Carbs: 8g | Protein: 9g

Conclusion

The technology of this Smart Oven is exceptionally straightforward. Fried foods get their crunchy feel because warm oil heats meals quickly and evenly onto their face. Oil is a superb heat conductor that aids with simultaneous and fast cooking across each ingredient. For decades' cooks have employed convection ovens to attempt and mimic the effects of cooking or frying the entire surface of the food.

However, the atmosphere never circulates quickly enough to precisely attain that yummy surface most of us enjoy in fried foods. With this mechanism, the atmosphere is spread high levels up to 400°F, into "air fry" any foods like poultry, fish or processors, etc. This technology has altered the entire cooking notion by decreasing the fat by around 80 percent compared to traditional fat skillet. There is also an exhaust fan directly over the cooking room, which offers the meals necessary airflow. This also contributes to precisely the identical heating reaching every region of the food that's being cooked. This is the only grill and exhaust fan that helps the Smart Oven improve the air continuously to cook wholesome meals without fat. The inner pressure strengthens the temperature, which will be controlled by the exhaust system. Exhaust enthusiast releases filtered additional air to cook the meals in a far healthier way. Smart Oven doesn't have any odor whatsoever, and It's benign, making it easy and environment-friendly.

Hopefully, after going through this cookbook and trying out a couple of recipes, you will get to understand the flexibility and utility of the air fryers. The use of this kitchen appliance ensures that the making of some of your favorite snacks and meals will be carried out in a stress-free manner without hassling around, which invariably legitimizes its worth and gives you value for your money.

We are so glad you leaped this healthier cooking format with us!

The air fryer truly is not a gadget that should stay on the shelf. Instead, take it out and give it a whirl when you are whipping up one of your tried-and-true recipes or if you are starting to get your feet wet with the air frying method.

Regardless of appliances, recipes, or dietary concerns, we hope you have fun in your kitchen. Between food preparation, cooking time, and then the cleanup, a lot of time is spent in this one room, so it should be as fun as possible.

This is just the start. There are no limits to working with the air fryer, and we will explore some more recipes as well. In addition to all the great options that we talked about before, you will find that there are tasty desserts that can make those sweet teeth in no time, and some great sauces and dressing to always be in control over the foods you eat. There are just so many options to choose from that it won't take long before you find a whole bunch of recipes to use, and before you start to wonder why you didn't get the air fryer so much sooner. There are so numerous things to admire about the air fryer, and it becomes an even better tool to use when you have the right recipes in place and can use them. And there are so many fantastic recipes that work well in the air fryer and can get dinner on the table in no time.

We are pleased that you pursue this Air Fryer cookbook.

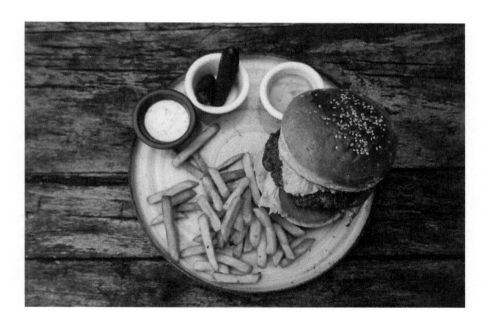

If you enjoyed this cookbook
don't miss this bonus designed for our readers

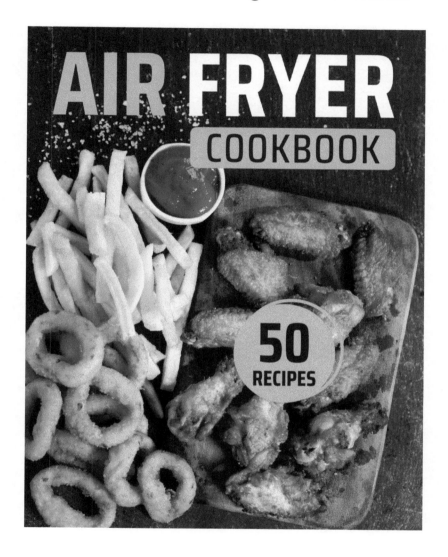

DOWNLOAD FOR FREE
www.getYourAirFryerRecipes.com

Lightning Source UK Ltd.
Milton Keynes UK
UKHW020842040621
384920UK00001B/67